T0169551

7 CAREGIVER LANDMINES

7 CAREGIVER LANDMINES

And How You Can Avoid Them

PETER W. ROSENBERGER

NEW YORK

LONDON • NASHVILLE • MELBOURNE • VANCOUVER

7 CAREGIVER LANDMINES
And How You Can Avoid Them

© 2019 Peter W. Rosenberger

Published in New York, New York, by Morgan James Publishing. Morgan James is a trademark of Morgan James, LLC. www.MorganJamesPublishing.com

The Morgan James Speakers Group can bring authors to your live event. For more information or to book an event visit The Morgan James Speakers Group at www.TheMorganJamesSpeakersGroup.com.

ISBN 978-1-64279-001-6 paperback
ISBN 978-1-64279-002-3 eBook
Library of Congress Control Number: 2018935511

Cover Design by:	Interior Design by:
Rachel Lopez	Bonnie Bushman
www.r2cdesign.com	The Whole Caboodle Graphic Design

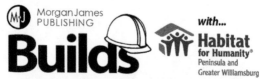

In an effort to support local communities, raise awareness and funds, Morgan James Publishing donates a percentage of all book sales for the life of each book to Habitat for Humanity Peninsula and Greater Williamsburg.

Get involved today! Visit
www.MorganJamesBuilds.com

TABLE OF CONTENTS

Introduction   *vii*

Landmine #1: Ignoring Personal Health   1
    Needs
Your Caregiver Minute: See Your Doctor   *8*
Landmine #2: Isolation   11
Your Caregiver Minute: Don't Believe   *18*
    Everything You Think
Landmine #3: Excessive Weight Gain   21
Your Caregiver Minute: The Goal Isn't   *28*
    To Feel Better, It's To Be Better
Landmine #4: Loss of Identity   31
Your Caregiver Minute: Discretionary   *37*
    Valor

Landmine #5: Guilt   39
  Your Caregiver Minute: The Amazing   45
     But Overlooked Attendance Record
     Of Caregivers
Landmine #6: Fear   47
  Your Caregiver Minute: Fight What's Closest   53
Landmine #7: "It's All Up To Me!"   55
  Your Caregiver Minute: Take Time for   65
     Stillness, Or Make Time for Illness
Bonus Chapter   67

About the Author   73
An Exceptional Voice of Experience for an   73
     Unprecedented Need
Other Items by Peter Rosenberger   77

INTRODUCTION

What does it feel like to be a caregiver?

It's kind of like coming to a road, looking both ways—and then getting hit by a plane!

For more than thirty years, I've been a caregiver for my wife through a medical nightmare that continues to bring new challenges—often daily. This journey shows no signs of slowing down. Along the way, I've had ample time to make virtually every mistake one can make as a caregiver.

Through this journey and through all the mistakes, I've also gained hard-won wisdom and experienced teachable lessons on the challenges, predicaments, and heartache of the caregiver. One of those teachable moments came following a snowmobile excursion in the forests of Montana with our youngest son, Grayson.

Ten miles from the paved road in a tiny town in Montana, my in-laws' home backs up to the national forest. No stranger to snowmobiles, Grayson and I headed into the mountains and traveled deep into the vast Montana wilderness one afternoon. Trails are marked by reflectors posted periodically on trees, and if you are not paying attention, it can be easy to miss one of those markers.

Although logging many hours on those trails, this day was a windy one, and the fresh snow covered any tracks made by previous riders. Speeding along the trail, I missed a marker. Finding ourselves on a slope, in a deep snow drift, my machine sank into the soft powder and quickly became stuck.

Getting a sled out of deep snow is not too bad if you have two people, but to complicate matters, we were lost. We'd have to work to get the machine freed and somehow make it back up the hill (in the soft snow) and find the marker. So, if we spent all our energy digging the machine out of the snow, we still ran the risk of getting stuck in an even worse place—unless we knew where the trail lay and could get our bearings there.

As we pondered our situation, the sun slowly sank over the peaks, and the temperature dropped. The wind howled, and snow whipped around us. I admit feeling more than a little unsettled. Not thinking about the house, not even thinking about five miles down the mountain, I simply wanted to find that next marker. The only goal was to navigate to a place of safety and get my bearings.

After a systematic search using Grayson's machine, which he kept away from the soft drifts, we found the marker. Then, we worked together to free my sled from the deep snow. With my heart racing, I gunned the machine, felt it take hold, and made a beeline for the marker and the trail—where I knew the packed snow would make it easier to navigate and provide a haven to catch my breath. Successfully feeling the packed snow of the trail, Grayson and I safely headed down the mountain.

Now, how does any of this relate to this book—and why was this a teachable moment for me as a caregiver?

As caregivers, we often find ourselves stuck in precarious circumstances, with deteriorating situations. Even if we spent the resources (money, energy, time) to get "unstuck," we don't often know where the path to safety lies, and we risk getting into an even worse spot—with fewer resources.

We need to find the marker and catch our breath.

As caregivers, we often can't think years, months, or even weeks down the road. All we can do is take the next right step, stay on a path to safety, and follow the markers to stay on a trail that is often hard to see.

In that snow-covered field, I couldn't simply walk around. The snow was so soft that I sank up to my waist at times and had to be careful where I stepped. Each time I floundered in the snow, I risked getting hurt, wasting precious energy, stepping into a covered hole, and even compromising the ability of my son to help me.

The road of a caregiver also has "landmines." Not actual explosives, of course, but beliefs and behaviors that cause serious damage to a caregiver, as well as to that caregiver's loved one. So not only do we need to know where the path to safety is, we need to know how to avoid those dangerous landmines that can cripple caregivers.

That's what this book is all about. In this book, we will discuss seven caregiver landmines that can wreak havoc in a caregiver's life—and the life of the caregiver's vulnerable loved one.

Despite all our skills, blinding speed, and apparent competency, all caregivers suffer from the same challenge: what we do is unsustainable. It's simply a matter of time before a caregiver's body, emotions, and/or wallet break down.

When caregivers recklessly hurl themselves at managing "that which cannot be managed," we rely on two things: our own abilities and the belief that we will outlive our loved ones.

Both beliefs create a serious risk of harming the very people we seek to serve. If the caregiver goes down, this has disastrous implications for the loved one who is already vulnerable.

Yet, we caregivers tend to "white-knuckle" through the brutal times—while taking physical and emotional "shortcuts" for our own health. On that snow-covered field, there were no shortcuts. There was only one path, and I had to think it through; look for the marker and then make a beeline for it. I knew the general direction of the house, but between me and that ten-mile expanse lay even more dangerous places. Consequently, the only way I could safely get off that mountain was to find the marker and get back on the trail.

I point caregivers to the next marker and help them make a beeline for safety. While the end of the trail for us as caregivers is uncertain, there is no doubt, however, that our loved ones will suffer even worse than they do now if we as caregivers are not in a safe and healthy place today.

One of the advantages of serving as a caregiver for as long as I have is that I've had ample time to make about every mistake possible as a caregiver.

The dark roads are familiar to me, and I recognize dead-ends and cul-de-sacs. And I've got the scars to prove my experience with caregiver landmines.

You don't have to get those scars—but even if you do have them, you don't have to keep getting injured by the same landmines.

Together, we can navigate to safety.

So, take a deep breath. Inhale for four seconds, and then slowly exhale for eight seconds.

See, you can immediately feel yourself calming down. (It's never helpful to hyperventilate when walking through a minefield!)

Okay. Ready? Let's begin!

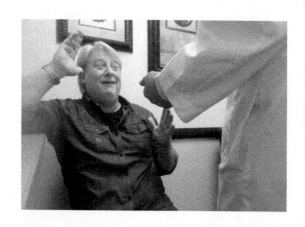

Landmine #1

IGNORING PERSONAL HEALTH NEEDS

I told the doctor I broke my leg in two places.
He told me to quit going to those places.
— Henny Youngman

There are 65+ million caregivers attending to the sickest in our country, and statistics show that 72% of us fail to see our own physician regularly.

Do the math, and "Houston …we have a problem!"

Caregivers see many doctors and often perform tasks previously relegated to licensed medical personnel. While those experiences teach us a lot about healthcare, the application of that knowledge for our own health is a different story. Most caregivers regularly take someone else to see a physician, but when was the last time we saw ours? We often grow so weary of taking others to a doctor's office that the thought of going to another one (or taking time off work …again!), well, it's just too much. Those "sandwich" caregivers caring for parents and their own family regularly feel stretched too painfully thin to carve out more hours for a doctor visit.

Many caregivers fear leaving their loved ones alone. Another justification used is that caregivers often don't have health insurance, and money is usually tight. I've heard every excuse and as a caregiver for three decades, I've given most of them. The reality doesn't change.

Regardless of the reasons WHY we don't see our own doctor, there are still two, nagging questions we caregivers must face:

- What good are we to our loved one if we stroke out, if we have heart disease, get diabetes, or some other malady?
- Who is in line to care for our loved one if we are out of the picture for a short-term illness, a long-term issue, or worse?

These two questions will persist into the national dialogue as the massive, baby-boomer population requires increasing care. Currently, a vast number of caregivers are already in the danger zone for their own health.

If I injure one of my feet, should I ignore it simply because my wife is missing both of her feet? Just because a cut toe pales next to her reality of double amputation doesn't mean I ignore the wound.

"Who am I to stop what I'm doing as her caregiver and attend to an injured foot—when she lost hers?"

That's the kind of reasoning we use as caregivers. We push our own health needs to the back burner. My feet are the only feet she can count on, and I need to be a good steward by properly caring for them. That principle applies across the board to our entire body (and hearts, wallets, jobs, etc.)

The first caregiver landmine is ignoring your own health needs as a caregiver. The dangerous shortcuts we give ourselves for this landmine are:

- There's no time to see my doctor.
- I don't have health insurance.
- When addressing my issues, I feel guilty.
- It's nothing compared to what she deals with.

Those shortcuts take caregivers into a dangerous place that can not only hurt them, but the loved one in their charge as well.

Serving as a caregiver can be brutal and requires extraordinary care for the caregiver. Caregivers can avoid this landmine by scheduling a medical professional to give the caregiver a once over—twice a year.

"Caregivers need an annual physical, and then six months later, a checkup for labs, blood pressure, etc. Why wait a whole year to discover high blood pressure, elevated sugar count, or other easily detected warning signs?"

Given the stress caregivers feel, it is critically important not to "sugar coat" it when meeting with your doctor. Your physician may instruct you to change your diet, exercise more, refer to counseling, or even prescribe medication to help with stress. Don't dismiss sound medical advice.

The primary care physician I've seen for nearly a dozen years watches me like a hawk, and I am grateful for him. Sometimes, with a minor ailment, I use a tele-medicine service which saves me hours and money. For a small monthly fee, I have unlimited access to a physician by phone/video for minor ailments, and there is a recording/transcript of the call to provide to my primary care physician. There is also an annual lab service as part of the subscription. The virtual doctor visits don't replace meeting with my physician, but it's another addition to the tool-belt of a caregiver that can help us live healthier lives.

Caregiving can be daunting and relentless. Those challenges sap the desire to fix a healthy meal, much less schedule time to go to yet another doctor visit. Yet that visit could very well save a caregiver's life. Caregiving can often feel like a full-contact sport, and is hard on the body, as well as the heart.

Make the call and keep the appointment for yourself as a caregiver. Doing so avoids the landmine of failing to treat the one body standing between your vulnerable loved one and an even worse disaster—yours!

Personally, I have always felt the best doctor in the world is the Veterinarian.

He can't ask his patients what's the matter.
He's just got to know.
> — **Will Rogers**

Your Caregiver Minute
See Your Doctor

Most caregivers regularly take someone else to see a physician, but when was the last time we saw our physician? We often grow so weary of taking others to a doctor's office that the thought of going to another one (or taking time off work … again!), well, it's just too much. Caregiving can be daunting and relentless. Those challenges sap the desire to fix a healthy meal, much less schedule time to go to yet another doctor visit. Yet that visit could very well save a caregiver's life.

Caregiving can often feel like a full-contact sport, and is hard on the body, as well as the heart. Make the call and keep the appointment for yourself as a caregiver. Doing so …. ensures treatment of **the one body** … standing between your vulnerable loved one and an even worse disaster—yours!

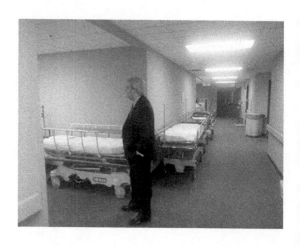

Landmine #2
ISOLATION

*Loneliness was the first thing that God's
eye named "not good."*
— **John Milton**

I n the Washington Post, a reporter recently
discussed a British survey of retired individuals
and the impact of social engagement on their
lifespan.

*But people who were members of social groups—
which could be a sports club, religious organization,
trade union or any other kind of leisure or professional
group — had a lower risk of death in the first six
years of retirement. Those who belonged to two groups*

before retirement and continued their activity in these groups had a two percent risk of death in the first six years. **Washington Post 2-16-2016**

This study affirms the positive impact of social connectivity on human lifespan, and going even further, on quality of life. Isolation is one of the most crippling long-term issues facing caregivers, and it leads to poor thinking, poor judgment, and poor behavior.

Pushing back against the isolation of caregiving is paramount for a caregiver. But where do you start?

In chapter one, we discussed the critically important first step of seeing a physician. That's as good a place to start as any. Having a medical professional seeing us as a caregiver opens the door to additional conversations—such as the need for support groups and counseling.

Furthermore, as caregivers, we need positive interaction. When, in our pushing back against isolation, we choose to hang around unhealthy individuals who bring us down emotionally or morally, we hurt ourselves.

In my book, HOPE FOR THE CAREGIVER, I tackled the subject of isolation and wrote the following:

> *Isolation often occurs due to logistics. Sometimes, it is not possible or practical for the caregiver to transport the loved one outside the home. Other times, caregivers, embarrassed about the condition of their loved ones, or wishing to protect their dignity, remove themselves from the public eye. There are many reasons for the isolation that caregivers feel, but the results are universally negative. Without positive human connections, everybody suffers. That's why it's important for caregivers to remain engaged in church, community, and other social networks. And, since caregivers can often feel lonely in a crowded*

room, it's important not only to attend but also to engage.
— From HOPE FOR THE CAREGIVER
©2014 Peter W. Rosenberger

I recently heard a great quote: "If you hang around five positive people, you will be the sixth. If you hang around five negative people, you'll be the sixth. If you hang around five idiots, you will be the sixth."

When we become isolated, our own dark thoughts take us down—often quickly. To best fight that, we need to surround ourselves with healthy, positive individuals. Sometimes it is as simple as a Facebook group, but that can only go so far. Regular phone conversations, regular face-to-face conversations, and when possible, group events, serve as the path towards pushing back against isolation.

We may have to start slow and not pin all our hopes on one individual, one phone call, or one encounter. Given that isolation often makes our hearts feel parched as if we have struggled through a hot desert with no water, we can be tempted to "guzzle" human contact. Any expert will tell you that when dehydrated, we need to sip water slowly and give our bodies a chance to hydrate properly.

The same thing applies to interaction. Let's don't make people "drink from the fire-hose" and hear every gruesome detail of our journey as a caregiver. Speaking slowly, deliberately, and calmly will ease us into a healthy engagement with others. Also, we can listen to others, as well.

The second caregiver landmine is isolation. Avoiding this landmine requires a deliberate action on our part to reach out to others. Here are three steps to take today.

1. Think of three people who you can trust. Pick up the phone and call them (one at a time …don't conference call! LOL). A heavy conversation isn't necessary—just "sip" the friendship slowly.

2. See a counselor. Whether a psychiatrist, psychologist, social worker, or licensed mental health counselor, it is critically important to involve a professional mental health expert in your journey.

3. Find a support group in your area. Maybe your doctor, pastor, or counselor can recommend one or simply look one up online. Virtually every disease or impairment has a support group attached to it, and you can find more by simply going online. If nothing is in your area, try going outside the box a bit and attend a local twelve-step recovery group. It may not be an exact fit for your specific situation, but you will still be listening to others share their journey in dealing with something they can't control. The goal is to be in community. Answers are often illusive or non-existent, but support, companionship, and the wisdom of others will strengthen

you—and allow you to help strengthen others. You may not be able to go as much as you would like, but you can go as much as you can.

Walking with a friend in the dark is better than walking alone in the light.
— **Helen Keller**

Your Caregiver Minute
Don't Believe Everything You Think

While physical isolation is one of the most challenging issues caregivers face, our thoughts become isolated, as well. In those lonely moments, our minds can play tricks on us, and take us down dark roads. Like a pilot flying through clouds without looking at instruments, we can quickly become disoriented. In those moments, we need external input ...an emotional GPS, if you will ...to help us regain our heading and proceed safely. We don't need to believe everything we think!

I don't know about you, but my mind is a dangerous neighborhood to walk in unaccompanied!

The Book of Proverbs tells us to trust in the Lord with all our hearts and to not lean on our own understanding. You know why that's in there? Because we lean on our understanding!!

Serving as a caregiver is simply too difficult to do alone. Don't lean on your understanding, ask for guidance and help. Don't believe everything you think!

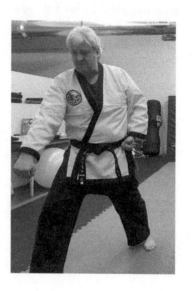

Landmine #3
EXCESSIVE WEIGHT GAIN

*My doctor told me to stop having intimate
dinners for four— unless there are three
other people.*
— **Orson Welles**

E ach of us know that excessive weight gain
harms our bodies and leads to all types of
physical and emotional challenges. When
you see someone who has rapidly put on
weight, or is thirty, fifty, or a hundred pounds
overweight—well, there's a reason.

During high stress times, cortisol (the stress
hormone) levels rise in our bodies. For caregivers,

"high-stress times" are daily. The stress we regularly encounter is nothing short of astonishing. Increased cortisol can lead to increased levels of insulin—which makes our blood sugar drop, and we crave a piece of pie rather than broccoli.

But that's not the only reason we look to food.

Think about it: an apple or doughnut? Celery or chocolate-chip cookies? Baked chicken with vegetables or lasagna?

There's a reason they call it "comfort-food," and in our culture, a measure of comfort is just a refrigerator away.

For many caregivers, making a sensible meal is simply another wearisome chore, and it's all too easy to swing through the drive-through.

That said, I see no need to create a caregiver diet plan that none of us will follow. We can leave it up to each of us to pick one of the countless meal planning options available to us from the experts. There's not a one-size- fits-all program for this landmine, and in my experience, this landmine doesn't originate in the kitchen, but rather in the heart.

Graham Kerr (known to the world as "The Galloping Gourmet") shared his journey from decadent food to heart healthy. Many don't know that Graham served as a caregiver for nearly thirty years. While caring for his wife, he changed the way he looked at food—then he changed the way he prepared each meal. His message to caregivers during an interview on my radio show was: "Make simple substitutions, and control portions." In doing so, we slowly, but effectively, incorporate a heart-healthy eating lifestyle. His simple message pointed us to the "marker" of a healthier approach to food—so we can avoid the landmine of excessive weight gain.

We're stressed. Weary and discouraged, we simply want comfort. Food, particularly fatty food, provides a temporary relief, but by indulging in food for relief, we ultimately harm ourselves further—and we do it with a knife and fork.

Like Graham Kerr, another friend of mine helps me with this. Rather than throwing a comprehensive plan at me, he shares an easy, helpful tip: "Make one simple change."

Maybe that change is to stop buying sodas. Okay. That's it.

Make that change. Let it take hold, and then watch the results. When that's settled in, make another change, and so forth. If we're overweight, we didn't get here overnight—and we won't lose the weight overnight, so let's manage the expectations and move slowly in the right direction.

Remember, however, the stress is real, and relentless. Even making one simple change, we still need to deal with that stress in a healthy manner. We can address our stress in several ways.

- Exercise (Joining a gym isn't required. Try just walking.)
- Counseling

- Meditation/Prayer/Quiet times
- Drinking lots of water

Again, we're going to start slow. We tend to put ourselves under more stress by trying to tackle another activity. Reducing our stress is not another task we need to accomplish and check off—rather, it's a lifestyle change.

Remember at the beginning of this book where I discussed taking a deep breath, and then exhaling twice as long as you inhaled? There is no faster way to bleed off stress than to learn to properly breathe.

By the way, breathing is free.

If we choose to participate in activities that are healthy and calm us down, it will lesson our desire to graze. Once we're in a calmer frame of mind, we can tackle pushing ourselves a bit to exercise more and participate in healthier activities.

For me, I do martial arts. I'm working on my third-degree black-belt as I write this. In addition,

I'm a pianist so I take time to sit at the piano and musically work out the kinks in my soul. (Also, it's hard to eat a piece of cake while both hands are on the keyboard!)

Gardening, painting, crafts, golf, hiking—whatever it is that speaks to that stressed-out place in your heart, give yourself permission to do it regularly.

Someone once asked me, "How do you find time to do the things you do?"

I don't FIND time to do it. I MAKE time to do it. But it all starts with learning to be still and settle my heart down. I learned the hard way that if I don't take time for stillness, I will have to make time for illness. Calmness facilitates better decisions for the body.

The third caregiver landmine is excessive weight gain. Avoiding this landmine starts with redefining how we view food. It's fuel not comfort. The stress we feel cries out for relief. But it's not our bodies screaming for it—it's our heart.

Nothing in the fridge, pantry, or drive-through speaks to the needs of our weary hearts.

Make one simple change of what we eat once a week— or even once a month—at a time. As we make that change, we can also choose to participate in appropriate activities that help bleed off that stress. Making simple, healthy choices, step by step, will lead to those pounds slipping off.

You may discover, however, that the excessive weight you carry is not just around your waist, but in your heart.

That's the weight that needs to come off first.

- I got so big—it took TWO dogs to bark at me!
- I got so big—I was standing on a street corner and a cop told me to break it up!
- I got so big—I wore a yellow rain coat and kids thought I was the school bus!
- I got so big—I broke my family tree!

Your Caregiver Minute
The Goal Isn't To Feel Better,
It's To Be Better

As caregivers, we are weary, fearful, wounded souls trying to stand between a vulnerable loved one and even harsher circumstances. But the grim things we face can cause our hearts to daily break …and we cry out for relief …and to feel better. During our journey as a caregiver, there will be many times where we won't feel better. Someone we love suffers …and we're often powerless to do anything about it …you never feel better about that. But that's not the goal. The goal becomes to BE better as we journey through this often …long… valley of the shadow of death. To be healthier …on every level. Physically, emotionally, financially, spiritually. We can be healthy while caring for someone who isn't … Even if we feel heartbroken over what we must do as caregivers. We're not going to always feel better, but we can be better ...and let's do this together!

HELLO
MY NAME IS

Landmine #4
LOSS OF IDENTITY

This above all—to thine own self be true.
Polonius to Laertes, HAMLET Act I, Scene 3
— **William Shakespeare**

A friend's wife suffered through a rough couple of years with cancer, and he served as her sole caregiver.

Meeting up with him one day, I asked, "How are you doing?"

He quickly replied, "Well, we're doing okay. She just got home from the hospital and seems to be having some better days. We have a long way to go, but our situation is better than it

31

was." He then shared his wife's recent medical test results and provided a comprehensive update on her condition. After he paused for a moment, I pointedly said to him, "I asked how you are doing."

The ease of speech used to relay his wife's circumstances instantly vanished. As tears welled in his eyes, he managed to stammer, "Peter, I'm scared and worn out."

Both responses my friend gave me reflect the condition of virtually every caregiver I know—including myself.

We tend to lose our identity in the story of someone else. When a caregiver answers direct questions in third person singular (he, she, etc.) or first-person plural (we, our, us), it's a good indicator the loved one overshadows the caregiver's identity. When asked about our own hearts, however, we find ourselves caught off guard and usually struggle to share our feelings.

The fourth caregiver landmine is the loss of identity. It's simply too easy to become lost as the person pushing the wheelchair, the one standing in the hospital room corner, the one doing laundry or meals, etc. How can we talk about our own broken hearts or weariness when our loved ones have such drastic illnesses or challenges?

Too many caregivers feel guilty for saying anything construed as complaining or wanting a break—after all, the suffering loved one doesn't get a break from pain/disease/disability. But our injuries and wounds, whether physical or emotional, require attention—regardless of how they compare to others.

If we don't start paying attention to and taking care of ourselves, a strong resentment can quickly take hold. In a relatively short time, we can find ourselves tied in all kinds of emotional knots of guilt and other negative feelings. Most don't understand that caregivers can easily lose their identity in caring for that loved one—and it becomes hard to speak from their own hearts, pain, anger, frustration, and sadness.

This loss of identity is the first step on a downward spiral for a caregiver. Oddly, understanding this truth didn't come from counseling or support groups (both of which I recommend), but rather I learned this one at the piano.

Playing the piano since age five, I eventually earned a degree in music. While in college, I met Gracie who, although hurt from her terrible accident, is a wonderful singer. I mean, a no-kidding singer!

For years, we performed together, and I accompanied her on countless stages and in the studio. When Gracie's health declined, and she could no longer maintain a regular public schedule, my public performing appeared shelved as well.

My pastor, however, asked me to play before church services each Sunday morning as people gathered and help facilitate a more reverent atmosphere in the sanctuary prior to beginning of the service. Sitting down to play hymns I've played since childhood, I realized my wife's voice carried a residual impact. Within just a few measures, I discovered my playing left out the melody, and I played only the accompaniment. The chords were nice, but they didn't communicate the song. I had to train myself to play the melody.

This is where we caregivers often find ourselves: we lose the melody. Growing accustomed to someone else's voice, we find ourselves playing a supporting role.

The loss of our own voice, our melody—our identity, is a landmine with disastrous effect. That's why I spend so much time on this issue for my fellow caregivers.

We avoid this by reclaiming our identity and acknowledging our feelings out loud. Using our own voices, we can express, "I'm tired," "I'm lonely," "I'm scared," "I'm angry," or "I'm weary," and then seek (and receive) the help we need.

Caregivers can also reclaim healthy identities by cultivating trusted and appropriate relationships. In those relationships, caregivers can safely express feelings and challenges with someone who understands their needs. Not limited to just friendships, a relationship with a trained mental health counselor can help sort through the issues and even connect to various respite and similar community services.

Although each of these remain critical steps, they all start with a caregiver uttering: "I need help."

The next time a trusted friend asks, "How are you?" it may feel strange at first but try and answer in first person singular. Appropriately sharing your own heartache and feelings is not self-centered; it is healthy—and healthy caregivers make better caregivers.

Your Caregiver Minute
Discretionary Valor

When someone we love is hurting, suffering, or is impaired, we often leap to action and fight the danger. While a good trait in an emergency, it's unsustainable in the marathon of caregiving—particularly in relationship dynamics. That impulse to conquer a problem not only exhausts us, it can simultaneously engage us in way too many battles on multiple fronts.

As Don Diego stated to Alejandro in The Mask of Zorro, "Oh, yes, my friend, you would have fought very bravely, and died very quickly."

While bravery and action remain important, **discretionary valor** is equally, if not more, essential as a caregiver. That discretion of knowing when to act, speak, or be still—comes with time and practice …but it's an important part of our journey in becoming healthy caregivers. And healthy caregivers make better caregivers.

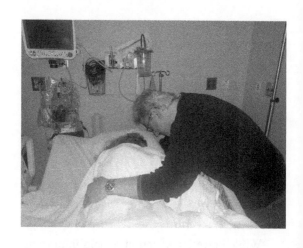

Landmine #5
GUILT

There's no problem so awful, that you can't add some guilt to it and make it even worse.
— **Bill Waterson**, The Complete Calvin and Hobbes

For every caregiver, guilt remains a seemingly insurmountable obstacle standing between us and a measure of peace in our hearts.

In the face of overwhelming odds, we put ourselves in an often-impossible situation, and keep doing it armed with little else than love—while spending blood, sweat, and treasure.

Yet with all that, we caregivers treat ourselves mercilessly—thinking somehow, through the lens of guilt, we must push ourselves to the breaking point.

I wouldn't hang around somebody who treats me the way I treat myself, and I'll bet you wouldn't either.

We've all heard the story of military drill instructors who look at a line of soldiers and ask for a volunteer. Then, everyone steps back—except the one guy who wasn't in on the planned exit. He didn't step back.

As caregivers, WE didn't step back. We show up every day. Sometimes we do it well—other times, we make mistakes. As caregivers, we sadly judge ourselves on our service record while completely overlooking our attendance record. We caregivers often harshly flog ourselves because we didn't do it as well as we think we should—or somebody else thinks we should.

We burden our already weary hearts with guilt.

This kind of caregiver guilt isn't about sins that get great press. Those things earn guilt.

Rather, this type of guilt comes from such things that weren't our fault, but we attribute blame to ourselves such as a child born with a disease or disability. Other times, we caregivers feel guilty over wishing the loved one would die— just so this painful journey would end.

We even torture ourselves with guilt over something as simple as wanting to take a break for a day—or even a few hours. The list of things we cruelly whip ourselves about is lengthy, but not one thing on the list helps us live a healthier life. We're no good to anyone if we stroke out or become impaired ourselves, because we allow guilt to push us to the brink.

A woman once called my radio show and expressed guilt because she didn't visit her mother at the nursing home every day.

Caring for her mother who struggled in the latter stages of Alzheimer's disease, this woman sank into despair each time she visited her. Yet if someone asked her about her mother, she'd berate herself internally if she failed to make an appearance at the home that day.

Listening to her for a few moments, I asked her a series of questions.

"Is she safe?" I inquired "Certainly," she responded.

"Is she cared for—clean, well-fed, warm?" "Absolutely!" She declared emphatically.

"Does she recognize the passage of time?"

"No."

"Does she know who you are?" "Sometimes."

"Can you be with her 24/7?"

"Of course not!"

"So, what you're telling me is, 'Your mother is being well cared for, and she doesn't always recognize who you are …and she doesn't know the passage of time, and you can't spend every moment with her, so I have two simple questions: How many breaks do you get …and who decides that number?"

[Silence]

After a hesitation, she stammered, "I never really thought of it that way."

Gently, I told her, "You've honored your mother and seen to her needs. It does not honor her, however, for you to become a husk of a person."

Even over the phone line to the radio studio, you could almost hear the stress melt off her as she realized she had needlessly placed such guilt on herself. Maybe for the first time, she allowed herself to acknowledge that she was doing the best she could with the brutal circumstances. Due to self-imposed standards, she had plenty of guilt, but little if any grace.

The fifth caregiver landmine is guilt. We avoid this landmine by appropriating another word to those feelings of guilt: Grace.

"Grace" is a beautiful word for caregivers to remember. To me, "Grace" is the loveliest name in the English language—I married a woman named Grace. I love saying her name.

As caregivers, we rarely give ourselves grace—to our detriment.

Healthy caregivers make better caregivers, and we cannot exist in a healthy state when carrying the crushing burden of guilt. It is okay, in fact, it is critical to our well-being, for us to extend grace to ourselves.

What would you say to friends doing exactly what you do? Would you criticize them? Heck no! You'd hug them and give them a meal. Furthermore, you'd tell them how amazing they are!

"Love your neighbor as yourself" (Mark 12:31) implies that you love yourself. Loving ourselves doesn't mean narcissism—it means caring for and valuing the extraordinary life that we are...and have been given. Today's a great day to avoid that landmine of guilt and to give ourselves some kindness ...and grace!

Your Caregiver Minute

The Amazing But Overlooked Attendance Record Of Caregivers

All too often, caregivers judge themselves mercilessly over their performance. With a supremely critical eye, we berate ourselves, while also allowing others to do the same. If we choose to judge ourselves, however, let's at least be fair and judge ourselves … on the whole. For example, …our attendance record—which is nearly perfect. We keep showing up!

Yeah …sometimes we show up late, while often feeling battered and bruised. Sometimes we're swearing under our breath like Yosemite Sam did in the old Looney Tunes cartoons. But we still show up!!! What is that worth? It is certainly worth taking a moment to acknowledge the extraordinary commitment and resolve of caregivers …and that includes you!

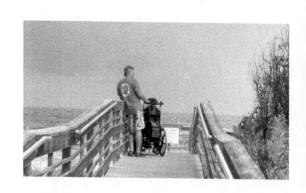

Landmine #6
FEAR

Angry people are fearful people and fearful people are angry people.
— **Unknown**

F or decades, my wife, Gracie, has suffered from "phantom-limb pain." Amputees can often feel the pain of a limb long since removed. An odd phenomenon, phantom-limb pain serves as another astonishing example of the complexity of the human body.

In kind of a "reverse phantom-limb pain," caregivers often feel pain—not over something missing, but rather something that hasn't even happened. We feel what we fear, and often don't see a positive end, but rather see it getting worse. Fretting over "what will happen if ..." adds despair to already weary hearts over something that hasn't occurred—or may never happen.

Years ago, a surgeon grimly returned to the hospital room where I waited for news from yet another surgery. He shared with me that Gracie contracted an infection in her back that required her to stay three months in the hospital, flat on her back (raising no more than 15 degrees). In addition, she would need an operation every third day to irrigate the infection site.

Thinking about Gracie, our young sons, my job, and all the things involved, my heart sank, and I mumbled, "I can't do this for three months."

Putting his hand on my shoulder, he said, "You're not going to do this for three months—you're going to do it for 24 hours. 'Tomorrow will worry about itself.'"

That event's lesson taught me (albeit with frequent reminders): today has enough drama, heartache, and challenges—I don't need to borrow any from tomorrow, three months from now, or thirty years from now. There is no need to indulge in pain that isn't there.

The sixth caregiver landmine is fear. The Bible tells us that "…fear hath torment" (I John 4:18 KJV). Fear paralyzes us. Fear can also incite us to rage and reactive behavior. Caregivers often see our money, our jobs, our independence, our health, and our very identity being sucked into the dark void of caregiving—and it frightens us.

We've all heard of the "Flight or Fight" adrenaline rush that comes at a crisis and felt it at one time or another. Caregivers, however, deal with relentless crises. Those waves of crises wash over us without mercy and usually at the worst times. They plunge us into what often feels like terror.

Constantly living in "Flight or Fight" is unsustainable as a caregiver, and it will eventually destroy us.

Caregiver stress wreaks enough havoc on our bodies and heart without us adding to it by living in the wreckage of our future. Letting our imaginations run wild with all sorts of things that may happen spikes our stress levels to staggering heights. The landmine of fear devastates caregivers.

Each day often brings an opportunity to race with fear, and its frequent companion: rage. But we are not doomed to those behaviors. Each day can also offer the opportunity to respond rather than react.

A martial arts instructor recently shared in a training seminar, "Fight what's closest—not what's beyond our reach." Applying that simple instruction to my role as a caregiver helps avoid the landmine of fear by living in the present and dealing with the reality at hand. I'm learning to accept what I can control, as well as what I can't.

*Quod si levior metus instat periculum
(A person's fears are lighter when the
danger is at hand)*
— **Lucius Annaeus Seneca**

Living in the present doesn't mean we can't
plan—nor does it mean that unpleasant things
aren't lurking just out of our vision. We're not
irresponsible, in denial, nor are we fatalistic.
Rather, we avoid the fear landmine by choosing
a path of doing what we can do—about what we
do know.

*Do what you can, with what you have,
where you are.*
— **Theodore Roosevelt**

As caregivers, real "fear-worthy" issues
regularly assault us. We don't, however, have to
go "toe-to-toe," gripped in mortal combat with
every issue. Side-stepping a few of those issues,

we can let go of the burning compulsion to obsess on them. Borrowing from my martial arts instructor, if we see an enemy on the horizon, keep an eye on that enemy—but deal with what is within arm's reach.

Responsibly, we do the next right thing, and learn to fight what's closest. We have enough danger and challenges today. Tomorrow will take care of itself.

> *Therefore do not be anxious about tomorrow, for tomorrow will be anxious for itself. Sufficient for the day is its own trouble.*
>
> **— Matthew 6:34**

Your Caregiver Minute
Fight What's Closest

Sometimes as caregivers, we look at the problems in our field of view and subsequently try to tackle all of them at once. The healthier approach is dealing with what is nearest to us. My martial arts instructor often tells me to "Fight what's closest!" A distant opponent can wait until we deal with the obstacle directly in front of us. Difficult things may lurk on the horizon for caregivers but fixating and fretting over them is unhealthy. Planning is appropriate, but we better serve ourselves and others by focusing on what lies within our grasp, rather than living in the wreckage of our future. Sometimes it's as easy as just doing the next right thing ...which may be taking a nap, calling a friend, or even visiting your own doctor. Look, we know that more challenges await us, but let's deal with today ...what's closest ...and do the next... right... thing.

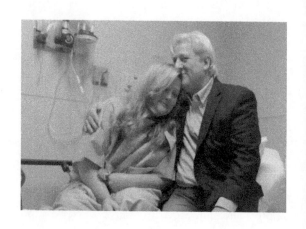

Landmine #7
"IT'S ALL UP TO ME!"

You just call out my name, and you know where ever I am I'll come running to see you again.
— **James Taylor**

We caregivers tend to hurl ourselves recklessly at caring for a vulnerable loved one—and assume the entire burden of their wellbeing on our shoulders.

Even as I wrote that statement, I had to let it sink into my own heart. This isn't theory to me—it is everyday life. Looking back over my three decades of this, I see where that belief system of

"It's all up to me!" took me into some unhealthy places—emotionally, physically, financially, and professionally. I still fight against that belief.

Many people mistakenly believe that the hot-button issues for caregivers are medical insurance, the medical community, family members, the loved one, and/or the chronic tasks—all of which weigh heavily upon us as caregivers. The relentless onslaught of crises, the "death by a thousand paper cuts," and the "valley of the shadow of death" stretching beyond the horizon—all those things can and do wreak havoc on a caregiver's well-being.

A lifetime of caregiving has convinced me, however, that the main issue for me as a caregiver is a relationship issue—but it is the relationship I have with myself. My heart, my beliefs, my reactions to events, my behavior and choices have all caused far greater stress than anything my wife's condition has ever done.

I don't have to wake up every day and ask someone else what kind of day I'm going to have!

Serving as caregiver, doesn't require me to feel miserable. In fact, I'm as miserable or as happy as I choose to be. Even while dealing with harsh realities, I don't have to be harsh—with others or with myself.

I spent a lifetime reacting to things beyond my control and trying to wear the superhero costume and run to the rescue—only to crash and burn in the face of something I remain powerless to change. As the "crash-test dummy of caregivers," I have arrived at a place in life where I'm comfortable stating what doesn't work—I've butted my head against enough walls to identify dead-ends, traps, and landmines for caregivers. Three decades provides ample time to make virtually every mistake possible as a caregiver.

And the biggest mistake is thinking that it's all up to me.

Once I better understood my role and responsibilities, I started to make healthier decisions. Making healthy decisions doesn't mean

I feel better about all this. In fact, I've learned that the goal is NOT to feel better. My wife is missing both legs, has endured so many surgeries, so many doctors, so many bills, and is in relentless pain—I'm NEVER going to feel better about any of that.

But I can be better as I care for her.

My role is one of stewardship—not ownership. I didn't do this to her, and I can't undo what has happened to her. But I can care for her to the best of my abilities—and part of caring for her is recognizing that I am only human and cannot …and must not …think that it's all up to me.

Asking for help is not a sign of weakness or defeat, but rather one of wisdom. Once we as caregivers accept that premise, then we can make additional healthier choices.

Looking in the eyes of countless fellow caregivers, I see past the weariness and encounter such strength of will, resolve, and self-sacrifice. We caregivers, quite bluntly, are an amazing group of people. We shoulder the impossible, attempt the unattainable, and try to manage the unmanageable—all out of love and a reflection of our own sense of duty and responsibility.

All that nobility, love, sacrifice, and character, however, can crash on the rocks of reality—we simply cannot sustain efforts at a consistent level of intensity.

We need help in every area of our lives.

- Health
- Emotions
- Lifestyle
- Profession
- Money
- Endurance

I put them in that order to spell out: HELP ME. Boiling it all down, crying "HELP ME" is the first step toward improving your life as a caregiver. Individuals in trouble rarely get better without asking for help.

As a frightened young man faced with a nightmare, I did not know how to ask for help—or maybe I asked for help but not in a way that others could understand. Every caregiver struggles with asking for help—usually due to at least one of the following reasons:

- Guilt
- Embarrassment
- Shame
- Not knowing what help looks like
- Being afraid of asking for help ...and being refused
- Being afraid of asking for help and the person doing it wrong—creating a bigger mess
- Being afraid of the person helping for a season and then simply quitting

Regardless of why we won't ask for help, it doesn't negate the fact that we need help.

If you go down, what happens to the individual(s) depending upon you? How will that vulnerable person function if your finances, emotions, and health all crash? If you lost your job today, how well would your caregiving system function?

As to the person you are caring for, I appreciate their pain, challenges, situation, and/or disability; it's serious and it's significant. They will, however, be in even more difficult circumstances if you are not functioning as a healthy individual. Emotionally, physically, spiritually, financially, professionally—each of these areas require constant attention.

Caregivers often fail to address these areas out of some misplaced ideology. Thinking that it's all up to us, we "white-knuckle" ourselves through this and often make unhealthy decisions in the isolation of our mind. We hit one or more of the seven caregiver landmines.

As caregivers, we do not have the ability to fix what our loved one endures. Yet we push ourselves to insane levels to manage something that is unmanageable. It's like rearranging deck chairs on the Titanic—we may look busy, but are we doing something that is sustainable?

Understanding our limitations changes our decision path. Our way becomes clearer towards asking for and receiving help.

Yet help is not necessarily getting more assistance for our loved ones—it's getting aid for us. As caregivers, we stand between our loved one and even worse things than they already fight. Our well-being directly affects theirs.

The seventh caregiver landmine is thinking that it is all up to us. We avoid this landmine by admitting and respecting our limitations. This landmine can also be avoided by raising our hand to ask for help.

Sometimes help is needed to accomplish a simple task, like cleaning the gutters or picking up groceries. Other times, it's asking someone to sit with our loved one while we go to the doctor for our own health needs. On even different occasions, help is needed in matters of the heart. In those times, we can ask a friend to listen to us, or we spend time with a clergy member or a mental health provider.

A common objection is, "I can't afford to pay for help." Upon digging deeper into that objection, the underlying belief is "I have to pay for help." That belief means it's still "all up to me."

The goal is not to map out the "how." The goal for us as caregivers is to admit the truth: "It's not all up to us."

Help may not come in the exact way we wish, but that's okay—we're still heading towards the marker when we ask for help. Over time, we will learn to fine-tune the request, but it starts with recognizing it's not all up to us and asking for assistance. Some may reject our request—that's okay, as well. A "no" is one step closer to a "yes."

I've discovered that it's often not a lack of resources, but rather a lack of resourcefulness. There are resources available. Maybe not the exact ones we desire, but ones that can move us further down path of healthy decisions. We didn't get here overnight, and we're not going to move past this overnight.

But we can make progress. Regardless of how many landmines we hit last week—or even yesterday, we don't have to hit the same ones today. We can look to those trail markers to help us regain our bearings, and we can start making healthy decisions today.

Healthy caregivers make better caregivers— and today is a great day to start being a healthy caregiver!

Your Caregiver Minute
*Take Time for Stillness,
Or Make Time for Illness*

Noise bombards us every day. From 24-hour cable news, to traffic, to our mobile devices, we are inundated with a wall of noise that seems to keep so many of us in a state of agitation. For caregivers, taking a moment to sit quietly and settle our hearts down …seems nearly impossible …but it's critical for us to do just that.

You see, if we don't take time for stillness …we're going to have to make time for illness. The constant state of anxiety, stress, and sensory overload we experience as caregivers will eventually make us sick. Stress kills. The way we push back on this ….is to carve out some time where we can just be still and quiet. Prayer, meditation, or just clearing our frenetic thoughts …it all helps re-boot our minds and hearts …and allows us to be a little calmer in the caregiver storm we navigate.

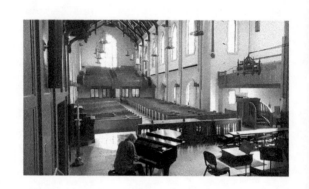

BONUS CHAPTER

Each of the landmines discussed in this book will hurt us. Left unaddressed, that hurt can lead to deep resentments which further compromise our ability to lead healthy lives and serve as healthy caregivers. The difficult challenge of resentment felt by caregivers inspired me to add this short chapter.

You Can't Play A Piano With Clenched Fists!
Caregivers and Resentment

Resentment seems to be a regular companion for caregivers. Often stemming from a deep-seated belief of obligation, caregivers drive themselves mercilessly with such internal commands such as, "I have to, I must, I'm supposed to, and I need to ..." In addition, all too many caregivers allow others to reinforce these beliefs as they become emotional punching bags from family, friends, their loved ones, and even the medical community. It can often seem that everyone in a caregiver's circle feels a need to critique a caregiver's job performance—and, sadly, the most vocal critics rarely help at all.

Is it any wonder that so many caring for the sickest among us feel beaten down and discouraged? These negative feelings cannot be suppressed or contained and will come out—usually in the form of resentment. In flash points, when caregivers feel presumed upon, undervalued, and unappreciated, that resentment forces its way to the surface. Once there, it creates an emotional mess that usually cripples the caregiver far more than it negatively affects others.

> *Nothing on earth consumes a man more completely than the passion of resentment.*
> —**Friedrich Nietzsche**

Struggling through my own caregiving journey, a teachable moment about resentment presented itself in an unusual place. A pianist for even longer than my three decades as a caregiver, I often find myself at the keyboard working out the kinks in my soul. Sitting at the piano, I discovered, however, that the music won't come if my fists remain clenched with resentment. Something beautiful flowing from my hands and heart requires opening both, along with a willingness to let go of resentment.

Each time my hands open to play something expressive and beautiful on the piano, it signals to my heart that it's okay to release grudges, slights, or bitterness. While maintaining healthy boundaries between my heart and those who either inadvertently or intentionally trample it, I can let go of the resentments. It's not easy, but the music flowing from that decision is soothing and healing to my soul—as well as to listeners.

Forgiveness doesn't mean it's unimportant. It simply means we're willing to take our hands off someone else's throat. Sometimes, the person we harbor the most resentment towards is our self—and we cruelly demean our own hearts for allowing us to either get into the circumstances we find ourselves, or for staying in the situation. Regardless of the targets of our resentment, it only serves to eat at our own peace of mind and well-being. We serve ourselves (and others) better when we live in a calmer and healthier manner, free of resentments and bitterness.

We all possess the ability to make and enjoy beautiful music and art in our own ways. As caregivers, that beauty is not limited by the harsh circumstances we face and carry, but rather limited only by our unwillingness to let go of resentment.

I picture myself at some point standing at a grave. While I can't guarantee outliving my wife and ensuring she and our sons aren't left to deal with her massive medical challenges without me, I can, however, guarantee a better chance of doing so if I live a healthier life. Part of living a healthier life is avoiding carrying resentment. I don't want to stand at that grave with clenched fists while feeling resentful at her, others who didn't help the way I wanted, myself, or at God.

Sitting at the piano I've played for a lifetime, I discovered that letting go of resentments often starts with the simple act of opening one's hand. The heart will follow.

And forgive us our debts, as we also have forgiven our debtors.
—Matthew 6:12

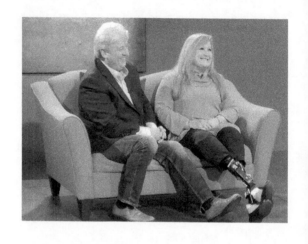

*Yea, though I walk through the valley of
the shadow of death,
I will fear no evil: for Thou art with me;
Thy rod and thy staff they comfort me.*

— **Psalm 23:4**

ABOUT THE AUTHOR

An Exceptional Voice of Experience
for an Unprecedented Need

For the past 30 years, radio host, author, speaker, pianist, and black-belt in Hapkido, Peter Rosenberger has personally traveled the path of the family caregiver. In the process, he has learned that a caregiver cannot only survive, but thrive in the midst of oftentimes grim circumstances. In an unparalleled journey with his wife Gracie, he has navigated a medical nightmare that has mushroomed to 80 operations, the amputation of both of Gracie's legs, treatment by more than 80 doctors in 12 hospitals, seven medical insurance companies, and $10 million in medical bills.

This experience unquestionably qualifies him as an expert on caregiver issues and has made him a most ardent champion for the family caregiver. Peter brings an astonishing understanding of health care issues and a deep compassion for fellow caregivers. Seamlessly weaving frankness with his outrageous humor, Peter brings freshness, hope and laughter into the painful places of caregiving. He regularly speaks on a wide range of topics that include healthcare and finances, caregivers in the workplace, facing adversity, thriving as a caregiver, and family relationships.

Earning a Bachelor of Music from Belmont University, Peter is an accomplished pianist and composer—and often incorporates his expressive style of music into his presentations as he entertains, inspires, and challenges audiences from all walks of life.

Since 2013, he has carried his message of health and hope for the caregiver to the airwaves, hosting his own weekly show, called HOPE FOR THE CAREGIVER, broadcast from Nashville.

In 2017, HOPE FOR THE CAREGIVER became the first radio show for family caregivers to go into syndication.

Peter's book, HOPE FOR THE CAREGIVER is now in its fifth printing, and his blog, videos, and radio show inspire and strengthen caregivers around the world.

Since 2002, Peter has served as the president and co-founder of Standing With Hope, a non-profit Christian ministry with two program areas:

- A prosthetic limb outreach to amputees in West Africa
- An outreach to family caregivers through Peter's radio show and speaking events.

For More Information and Resources

Visit: www.caregiverswithhope.com

OTHER ITEMS BY PETER ROSENBERGER

Hope for the Caregiver

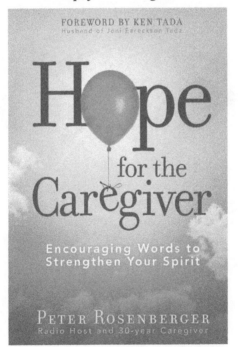

Songs for the Caregiver

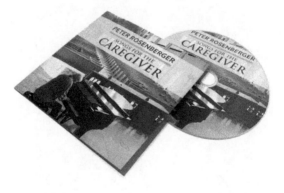

Foreword by Jeff Foxworthy

Gracie
standing with hope

GRACIE ROSENBERGER
as told to Peter W. Rosenberger

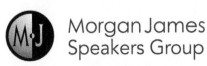

Morgan James
Speakers Group

We connect Morgan James published
authors with live and online events
and audiences who will benefit
from their expertise.

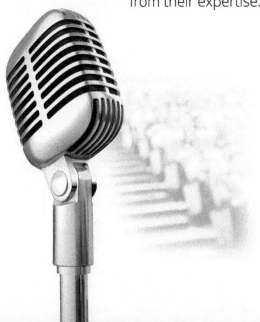

9 781642 790016